CONTENTS

INTRODUCTION **5**

COCKTAIL RECIPES **6**

Bloody Mary 7

Fruity 9

Gin And Ginger 10

Highball 11

Jack And Coke 11

Long Island Iced Tea 12

Margarita 14

Mojito 15

Moscow Mule 16

Mudslide 17

New Yorker 19

Orange Mango Rum 19

Orange Root Beer 20

Rum And Diet Coke 21

Rusty Nail 23

Sangria 24

Strawberry Daiquiri 25

Tequila Sunrise 26

Tropical Mango 27

Vodka Collins 28

White Russian 29

CHAMPAGNE COCKTAILS **31**

French 75 31

La Vie En Rose 32
Sparky Pepper 32
MIXERS 33
Sparkling Waters 33
KETO COCKTAIL RECIPES 35
Keto Margarita 35
Keto Cosmopolitan 36
Keto Mojito 37
Keto Moscow Mule 38
Keto Classic Daiquiri 39
Bourbon And Water 40
When To Add Water Or Ice To Whiskey 42
Scotch And Soda 44
Gin Martini 47
Customizing The Martini 51
Wine Spritzer 52
Best Wine For Wine Spritzers 54
Pickleback Shot 55
The Irish Whiskey 57
The Pickle Juice 58
Vodka Collins Cocktail 59
Separator Cocktail 62
Lemon Drop Martini 63
How To Create The Lemon Twist Garnish 67
Keto Hot Chocolate 68
Peppermint 71

Keto Eggnog ... 73
Raw Egg Warning ... 76
Low-Carb Raspberry & Blackberry Mojitos ... 78
Low Carb Margaritas ... 79
Low Carb Moscow Mules ... 80
Low Carb Sparkling Sangria ... 82
Vanilla Old-Fashioned ... 83
The Green Tox Cocktail ... 85
Low Carb Kamikaze Shot ... 86
Red Wine Berry Spritzer ... 87
Low Carb Lemon Drop Martini ... 88
Grapefruit Ginger Fizz ... 89

INTRODUCTION

James Bond has his martini - shaken, not stirred. In Casablanca they're drinking French 75s. Throughout the years, cocktails have called to our soul. During Prohibition they were drunk on the sly, sipped in the cellar. In modern times they're glitzy and wild, toasted in bars from Los Angeles to Tokyo There's just something about cocktails!

When you're embracing a low carb lifestyle, often it's tricky to know which cocktails are safe and which are simply loaded with sugar. It can be a challenge to keep track of which liqueurs are little more than sugar-syrup and which won't cause you to gain ten pounds with one sip.

I'm here to help!

Note that this is the first version of this book – it's got all my favorites in it. 24 recipes to be exact. If you've got a cocktail you adore that I don't have listed yet, contact me! I'm continually updating all of my low carb books. I'll be happy to investigate if we can create a low carb version of your cocktail, and then I'll add that to the next version of the book.

COCKTAIL RECIPES

Most hard liquors like rum, vodka, gin, and the like have zero carbs – but they *do* have calories. So they are a special case in low carb dieting. It's important to remember that your body burns alcohol as a fuel. Alcohol, being considered "toxic" by the body, is burned as quickly as possible. What this can mean is that by ingesting alcohol, anything else you eat does *not* get burned and instead gets stored as fat.

Here's an example. If you eat a steak on its own, your body burns those steak calories (from its protein) and uses them up. Your body doesn't store them as fat.

However, if you eat a steak while drinking an alcohol-filled cocktail, your body's first mission is to burn up that alcohol. It ignores the protein in a steak. You might then end up with that steak's energy being stored as fat.

A low carb diet assumes that you're not drinking alcohol. That's how the carb counting work. If you drink a lot of alcohol, then eating low carb won't keep you from gaining weight. Your body will gain weight based on the alcohol you ingest and the energy it's providing to you.

So, if your aim is to lose weight, go cautiously on the alcohol. It'll interfere with your weight loss. If you're maintaining, then drink in moderation!

Bloody Mary

If you're looking for a good 'scary' kind of drink for Halloween, the Bloody Mary would fit the bill nicely! It's tasty at other times of year as well, if you like a drink with a kick.

This cocktail is in essence spicy tomato juice and vodka.

Ingredients:

3oz tomato juice

1.5oz vodka

1/2 tsp Worcestershire sauce

2 drops Tabasco sauce

1 dash lemon juice

Shake all ingredients together with ice, and strain into a tall glass with ice cubes. Some people add salt and pepper.

I personally find this drink *very* salty - too salty to drink in fact. However, my mom loves these, so it is definitely a matter of each person having their own personal taste.

There is tomato juice with salt, and tomato juice without salt, so if you're on a low salt diet, you can go with the lower salt version.

Tomato juice has about 1.3g carbs per ounce, so for 3oz you are getting 3.9g of carbs. Call it an even 4 since people rarely measure out shots exactly. A bit more than wine per drink, but less than most beer.

If you're doing this for Halloween, get a plastic eyeball or two, and put them into your drink like ice cubes!

Who Was Bloody Mary

Bloody Mary was the nickname of Queen Mary I of England. She was only queen from 1553 to 1558. Her dad was Henry VIII and once she took control she actively tried to get the Roman Catholic church in control of England. Along the way she burned at least 300 of her enemies at the stake. She even killed the archbishop of Canterbury.

Desperate for a child to perpetuate her line, she married an enemy of the state, Philip II of Spain. This made her population even more upset with her. Her husband abandoned her, and she died only 5 years after she took control. With her death came in her sister, Elizabeth, one of the most famous monarchs in history!

Unfortunately, Bloody Mary never got to try this drink. It was invented in the 1920s in Paris, France, at the New York Bar. Fernand Petiot was the bartender who brought this cocktail to life.

Fruity

Looking for a cocktail that is low in sugars? This fruity combination of rum, vodka and sodas is 0g of carbs!

Ingredients:

1 shot vodka

1 shot rum

2.5 shots diet orange soda

2.5 shots diet lemon-lime soda

Put ice into a tall glass and mix in the four ingredients. This has got a great fruity flavor and 0g of carbs. Enjoy responsibly!

Be sure to avoid aspartame-sweetened diet sodas, look for those sweetened with Splenda instead.

Gin And Ginger

Looking for a delicious, low carb cocktail recipe? Gin and Ginger is a classic - simply make it with a Splenda-sweetened ginger ale!

1 part gin

4 parts diet ginger ale

splash lemon if desired

Put ice in tall glass, add in ginger ale. Stir in gin. Splash in lemon juice if desired.

I used the Waist Watchers citrus frost here because it comes with lemon flavors built in!

Carbs per serving: 0g

Highball

Back in the 1800s, the railway was the primary method of moving goods cross country. Millions of people worked on the railway. The Highball cocktail was invented as a quick recipe to entertaining these hard working people.

The drink was in fact named after the signal used when a train was moving through an area in a hurry.

By the 1920s, in cocktail-crazy gin joints around the world, the highball became a classic.

Ingredients:

2oz whiskey

diet ginger ale

Fill a tall glass with ice. Pour in 2oz of whiskey, then fill with ginger ale. Enjoy!

Jack And Coke

If you're on a low carb diet, a Jack and Coke is perfect - as long as you use diet Coke! When you do, this is perfectly zero carb.

Start with a tall glass of ice. Add in 2oz of Jack Daniels. Now fill the rest of the glass with Diet Coke.

Stir a bit, and enjoy!

Long Island Iced Tea

Long Island Iced Tea is a classic multi-alcohol cocktail that can be almost completely zero carb.

Just be sure to only have one! This is pretty much ALL ALCOHOL and is quite potent. Drinking in moderation is fun - drinking in excess can really be quite harmful to your body!

1/4oz gin

1/4oz rum

1/4oz vodka

1/4oz tequila

1/4oz triple sec

1oz sugar-free sour mix

dash diet coke

Put all into a shaker with ice and shake briefly.

Serve into a tall glass with lots of ice and enjoy!

Note that the ONLY item here with carbs in it is triple sec. Triple sec is an orange flavored liqueur. Triple sec has 12.5g of carbs per oz. If you "stepped up" to Curaçao which is also an orange flavored liqueur, that has only 10g of carbs per oz. Note this is still fairly steep, so of course an alternative is to make this without any orange liqueur at all.

Still, if you substitute in the Curaçao, that is only 2.5g of carbs since you're using only a quarter of an oz. For most people, even on induction, the 2.5g of carbs is doable in a healthy daily diet.

Even if you make it exactly as shown, then 1/4oz of triple sec is 3.1g of carbs per glass. Still not a big deal.

For those who are geographically challenged, Long Island is the long (go figure) island which is part of New York, but stretches out along beneath the state of Connecticut. It is famous for its many high end wineries, as well as mansions. The Great Gatsby novel was set on Long Island.

When my friend Kris and I biked around Block Island, which is near Long Island, we of course had to drink Long Island Iced Teas during our lunch stop.

Margarita

Most margarita recipes involve Curaçao, triple sec or Grand Marnier. All are LOADED with sugar. Here's a great recipe that is pretty much 0g carbs!

First, a little bit of background. Curaçao is a traditional Caribbean alcohol made with orange peels, grapefruit peels, rum, and a LOT of sugar. From that base are created other 'blends' such as triple sec and Cointreau. Grand Marnier is in essence a French version made with orange peels, sugar and brandy.

Ingredients:

1/2 tsp orange extract

1 packet Splenda (or 2 tsp powdered)

1 tsp water

1 shot tequila

1/8 tsp lime juice

1/4 tsp lemon juice

Mix together the orange extract, Splenda and water. This pretty much is the Curaçao - orange extract is up to 85% alcohol. Put crushed ice into a shaker and pour this liquid over the ice. Now add in 1 shot tequila, plus the lemon and lime juice. Shake thoroughly and pour into a glass.

You are practically at 0g of carbs here. You get a tiny amount of carbs (let's say 0.4g) from those dashes of lemon and lime juice.

Mojito

Mojitos are popular Cuban style drinks involving rum, lime and mint. These were made popular by James Bond, in the movie Die Another Day, but of course mojitos have been seen and enjoyed in many other movies and situations!

Here's how you can make a delicious, low carb mojito!

Start with a tall, thin glass. Take a fork, and using fresh mint leaves, press them around on the inside of the glass. 3-4 fresh leaves should do the trick.

Next, add in 2 tsp Splenda, and 3 Tbsp of lime juice. Stir this together. Dump in a lot of ice. Now comes the rum! Rum is zero carb. Finally, add in some diet club soda.

Garnish with a lemon slice if desired, and enjoy!

The only real carbs here are in the lime juice. You get about 5 1/2 g of carbs for standard lime juice, for those 3 Tbsp. On the other hand, there are low carb lime juices out there - if you love mojitos it may be well worth it for you to find out how to get your hands on some!

So mix up some mojitos, put on your favorite Bond movie, and enjoy!

Moscow Mule

The Moscow Mule is the classic vodka cocktail with a kick. Create it with a diet ginger ale to have a zero carb drink, perfect for the Atkins diet!

2oz vodka

1oz lime juice

diet ginger ale

Pour the vodka in over ice, add the lime juice, and top off with ginger ale.

I enjoy the flavored ginger ales, but the regular kind works fine as well.

Carbs per serving: 0g

Mudslide

Mudslides are delicious, creamy cocktails - and are also chock full of sugar. The sole reason they are high sugar is the Kahlua. Here is a way to make a mudslide cocktail without all of the extra sugar and carbs you would normally find in the drink.

First off, what is a mudslide? The basic recipe for a mudslide is –

1/2 ounce Vodka

1/2 ounce Kahlua

1/4 ounce Irish Cream liqueur

So, let's take this step by step.

First, the vodka. Vodka isn't a problem, it is straight alcohol. That is zero carbs.

The Kahlua IS a problem. Kahlua is a Mexican liquor that tastes like coffee. Kahlua has a massive 17g of carbs per 1oz shot. That's like downing liquid sugar! Here's the solution. A recipe for homemade low carb Kahlua is coffee, sugar, vanilla, vodka and brandy. We can use Splenda for sugar. Brandy and vodka are both 0g carbs. Vanilla is pretty much 0g at the amounts used. So is coffee.

To make the Kahlua, use:

1/4 cup STRONG brewed coffee

1/4 cup Splenda

1 tsp vanilla

4oz vodka

4oz brandy

Mix the coffee, Splenda and vanilla, then cool down to room temperature and add in the alcohols. The total is pretty much zero carbs. Irish Cream liqueur - i.e. Bailey's Irish Cream - is about 5.5g per ounce. So at 1/4oz, that's only about 1g of carbs. For me that's not worth fighting with, I can deal with my entire drink being 1g of carbs. If you really want to take a shot at making your own low carb Irish Cream, be my guest!

Shake all well with crushed ice, and strain into a glass!

New Yorker

This bourbon cocktail adds a splash of grenadine for color, and lime for flavor.

1 1/2oz bourbon

splash grenadine

splash lime

Pour all 3 ingredients over ice in an old fashioned glass.

Stir well.

Orange Mango Rum

If you like tropical, rum cocktails, this is a perfect sugar-free version that is really tasty! It's super easy to make, too.

Simply put 1 oz of rum into a tall glass with ice. Add in Sparkling Ice's Orange Mango to fill up.

Decorate and enjoy!

Orange Root Beer

Looking for a new flavor of cocktail to enjoy on your low carb diet? Just combine rum, orange soda and root beer, mix and serve!

1oz rum

1oz diet root beer

1oz diet orange soda

Mix all together in a glass and enjoy!

This is especially good for women, because it's a non-cola drink. For some reason Cola and other sodas containing phosphoric acid seem to cause soft bones in women – but not in men.

So if you're female, it's a good idea to avoid those colas and drink the other sodas instead!

Rum And Diet Coke

Rum and Coke was one of my favorite drinks in my 20s. Once I began eating more healthily, it was very simple to swap a diet Coke in for the regular sugar-filled Coke!

The ingredients here are rather simple –

start with a few ice cubes

add 1oz Rum

Fill glass with diet coke

garnish with a slice of lime

That's it! Remember to use *regular* rum in this - i.e. Bacardi rum or something like that. As soon as you start going for the flavored rums, you're introducing carbs.

Rum has zero carbs, and diet Coke has zero carbs. So this is a carb free beverage!

Note that this is also called a Cuba Libre. Cuba Libre literally means Free Cuba, and is a cocktail first drunk by revolutionaries in the 1900s. The Andrews sisters sang about Rum and Coca Cola, and it became popular!

The drink was originally mixed in the late 1800s down south. It was the time of the Spanish-American War and the US was helping Cuba gain its freedom. The American soldiers would mix together the local rums with the newly created Coca Cola. Coca Cola first came out in 1886 and had cocaine in it, so the idea of mixing together cheap-and-interesting Coke with cheap-and-intoxicating Rum was a great one.

Even so, the popularity of Cuba Libre was pretty low key until the Andrews Sisters came along. In 1944, in the midst of World War II and soldiers looking for fun amidst the fighting, they created the song "Rum and Coca Cola". An instant hit, it popularized the island drink for the entire world. Soon Rum and Cokes were being poured in every bar.

Rusty Nail

The Rusty Nail is a Scottish drink blending Scotch and Drambuie. This is a perfect low carb cocktail for fall / autumn drinking, with its golden brown color and hearty kick!

For those who are curious, Drambuie is a mixed liquor made in Scotland, and its name comes from the Gaelic phrase "the drink that satisfies". It is mostly Scotch whisky blends plus honey.

Drambuie has 9g of carbs, 0g fat and 439 calories per 30ml serving.

Really, Scotch Whisky (or Scotch for short) is just whisky made in Scotland. The flavor variation comes, as with wines and other handmade items, from the local ingredients used. In this case, it has to do with the Scotch waters, the peat used to cook the malt, and other similar idiosyncrasies.

To make a Rusty Nail, fill an old-fashioned glass with ice cubes. Pour in 3/4oz Scotch. Gently add the 1/4oz Drambuie. Depending on your taste preferences, you can also go with 1 shot Scotch and 1 shot Drambuie.

I suppose it depends if you have a really good Scotch that you want to appreciate, or if you want to drown out your mediocre Scotch with the honey in the Drambuie.

Sangria

Sangria is a light, fruity drink that's perfect for sipping. This easy recipe is low carb, perfect for Atkins and south beach dieters, and is quick to make!

Ingredients:

1 bottle red wine

1 bottle diet Orange soda

Put ice into a glass. Fill half the glass with red wine. Add the orange soda to fill. Enjoy!

1g per serving

Note that I keep a box of Cabernet Sauvignon in the fridge - it's really inexpensive per glass that way, and the wine is actually pretty tasty. For diet soda, we use the Waist Watchers brand, which has a wide variety of flavors all sweetened with Splenda. Try to stay away from those Aspartame-sweetened diet drinks!

Mix it up with different flavored sodas. If you're further along in your diet plan, or on maintenance, you might add in some hard liquor, fruits, and berries to the mix.

Strawberry Daiquiri

Bring a bit of island living into your life with this delicious recipe for a strawberry daiquiri. It's fresh and fruity, and best of all it's low carb too!

Ingredients:

8 strawberries

6 ice cubes

3 packets Splenda

2oz rum

1oz lime juice

Pull off the strawberries leaves and then core out the inner center of each. Drop all ingredients into a blender and blend until smooth. Serve with a tropical flair!

Strawberries are the only real carbs here, and they are only 1.8g per 1/4 cup.

Tequila Sunrise

This is one of the most beautiful drinks I know. A gorgeous sunrise of orange and red! Here's how to make a low carb version of the tequila sunrise.

Ingredients -

low carb orange juice

tequila

grenadine

First, mix two shots of tequila with orange juice and ice cubes.

Then pour 1/2 shot grenadine down the side of glass to the bottom. It will slowly rise up through the OJ in a very pretty color gradient from red to red-orange to orange.

When you use a low carb orange juice, you get **90%** less sugar than normal orange juice! And to think parents feed orange juice to their kids as a healthy drink. The low carb version is only 4g of carbs per glass. The tequila is zero carb, as is it an alcohol.

What about grenadine? Grenadine is an interesting topic. In short it's just ground up pomegranates. If you get the fake stuff, it's sugar water with red food coloring. So you either are getting fruit juice, or sugar water. It can be up to 5g if you go with the sugary variety.

Tropical Mango

Usually tropical drinks involve high sugar mixes such as Midori or Grand Marnier. Here's a great summertime low carb breezer to enjoy by your favorite beach!

Ingredients:

3 shots Mango Tropical Minute Maid

1/3 shot Bacardi 151 Rum

1/2 shot Bacardi Rum

1/4 tsp orange extract

1/8 tsp lime juice

Start with a tall, thin glass and fill it with ice. Mix in all ingredients and stir well. Top with an umbrella, and enjoy!

I really enjoy this cocktail, it has a gorgeous yellow-orange color, and a fresh citrus flavor.

This is pretty much zero carb, as long as you are using the diet Minute Maid of course! If you can't find that specific Minute Maid, then any tropical blend diet drink will do.

Vodka Collins

If you're a low carber, give a vodka collins a try. These cocktails are tasty and low carb too!

2oz vodka

1/2 oz lemon juice

1 tsp Splenda

carbonated water

Shake the vodka, lemon juice and Splenda with ice, then strain into a Collins glass. Fill up with carbonated water. You can add a slice of lemon for decoration and added flavor. Tradition is that you drink this with a straw!

A collins glass is really just a tall, thin version of a regular glass, which is known as a "highball" glass.

Vodka is zero carbs, as is Splenda and water. The only thing here with carbs is the lemon juice, 1.2g for the 1/2oz.

Because the vodka is not "hidden" by any other flavors here, it pays to get yourself a good quality vodka. It's like eating ice cream - if you're going to douse it in syrup and other things, it doesn't really matter what the ice cream tastes like. But if you're just going to eat it plain, as a special treat, it can be worth it to get something really tasty.

This is a great drink recipe in that all you really need is vodka. The rest of the ingredients are all common items you probably have lying around the house anyway.

White Russian

A White Russian is a creamy cocktail that has great flavors to it. It is, simply, a mix of Kahlua, vodka and milk. Luckily, you can make a quite low carb / low sugar version of this drink.

First, let me warn you that Kahlua has a massive 17g of carbs per 1oz shot. It is *full* of sugars. Milk can also be high in sugar in its natural state, up to 12g per 1 cup glass. Vodka has 0g of carbs, but you're already doomed with the other 2 ingredients.

Luckily, *coffee* is zero carb. In essence, a recipe for homemade Kahlua is coffee, sugar, vanilla, and brandy. We can use Splenda for sugar, and brandy is 0g carbs. Vanilla is pretty much 0g at the amounts used. So the key to making this a low carb recipe is to create your own Kahlua and use that.

Ingredients:

1/4 cup STRONG brewed coffee

1/4 cup Splenda

1 tsp vanilla

4oz vodka

4oz brandy

2oz (1/4 cup) low carb milk

Make your favorite coffee, but be sure that it's strong. Pour out 1/4 cup into a mixing bowl. Blend the Splenda and vanilla into this. Feel free to substitute in other sugar alternatives if you wish.

Next, cool this mixture down. You can do this quickly in the freezer, or toss some plastic ice cubes into it. Once it's cool (maybe 5 minutes or so) mix in the vodka, brandy and milk.

The brilliant part of this is you get maybe about 1g from the low carb milk, and that's really it! So you save a TON of carbs by making it yourself, plus it's far cheaper and yummier!

Carb Count: just figure out what 1/4 cup of your favorite low carb milk is, and that's it!

CHAMPAGNE COCKTAILS

I adore Champagne. It's important to note, though, that while most wine does not have sugar added to it, Champagne *does*. This added sugar is known as the "dosage" and it can vary based on the style of Champagne. So you could get anywhere from 5g to 10g of sugar in your glass, depending on how much Champagne you drink and if it's a sweet or dry (non-sweet) style.

It's fine to enjoy Champagne cocktails – just do so in moderation!

French 75

French 75s are famous cocktails that were even featured in Casablanca with Humphrey Bogart. A classic touch for any afternoon or evening!

1 shot gin

1/2 shot lime juice

1 tsp sugar substitute

Champagne

Shake the gin, lime juice and sugar sub with ice cubes. Strain and pour into a Champagne flute. Pour Champagne on top, and garnish with a lemon twist.

La Vie En Rose

The days of wine and roses are here. Sit back, relax, and find true romance in your life with this rose inspired drink.

1/2 shot glass rose water

1 tsp sugar substitute

Rose Champagne

If you don't have any rose water, it's easy enough to make. Get some rose petals - either from a rose in a florist shop or via the web. Wash them off. Add them into boiling water, then let it cool.

Mix the sugar substitute in the rose water. Put that into a flute glass. Rose Champagne is a pink colored Champagne made with red wine grapes. Add Rose Champagne into the glass until it's full. Add a strawberry as garnish, and toast!

Sparky Pepper

If you're a spice lover, this is the Champagne cocktail recipe for you!

1oz Absolut Peppar

Champagne

Absolut Peppar is an exotic concoction of vodka with paprika, chili, and green jalapeno peppers. Mix that in with a flute of Champagne, and spice up your world!

MIXERS

It's good to know the details about the mixers you use. Often you might think adding in a half-glass of orange juice creates a lovely color – but you forget about the enormous amounts of sugar this adds to the drink. Here are some details to be aware of when it comes to your cocktail mixers!

Sparkling Waters

Sparkling water, club soda, seltzer water, and the others. How do these differ from each other? Which are low carb? Which are healthy for you?

Let's start with the basics. Sparkling water is the generic, all-encompassing term for any water-based substance that is bubbly. It has gas injected into it to give it bubbles. So think of it as a flavorless, colorless, odorless soda. Bubbles, water, and nothing else. Sparkling water has zero calories and zero carbs. When I say "flavorless" I mean it doesn't taste like orange or grape or so on. Often water DOES have a gentle flavor to it, depending on its source.

The gas they tend to use for sparkling water is either hydrogen sulfide or carbon dioxide. Both are harmless. And some waters are naturally gas-filled, depending on where in the ground they have been sitting.

Next up is Seltzer Water. Seltzer Water is just sparkling water. This name comes from the German spring of Selters. So this was a natural, nothing-added sparkling water. It also has zero calories and zero carbs.

Soda Water or Club Soda is different. This is a sparkling water that has minerals added to it. It often has a sharp flavor. It can have sodium salts or bicarbonate of soda (baking soda) added to it. This will definitely add a flavor to whatever drink you're making to it. This is also zero calorie and zero carb.

Finally, we reach Tonic Water. With all the other water varieties having zero calories and carbs, people often mistakenly think this means they can pour in tonic water to their drinks and be home-free. However, that's not true! Tonic Water was created with quinine to help counter malaria. Now people enjoy its bitter flavor as a normal part of cocktail creation. And for a 12 ounce bottle of tonic water you can get 124 calories and 32g of carbs. So if you're aiming for a low carb lifestyle, you probably want to avoid tonic water for now.

So, to summarize, in most cases you'll do quite well with club soda, seltzer water, sparkling water, and so on. It's a great way to stay hydrated. Just try to avoid the tonic water.

KETO COCKTAIL RECIPES

Keto Margarita

Ingredients

1 jigger (1-½ ounces) tequila

2 tablespoons lime juice freshly squeezed

¼ cup water

¼ teaspoon orange extract

Ice

Optional: margarita salt or kosher salt

Optional: lime wedge for garnish

Allulose, erythritol or stevia sweeten to taste

Instructions

- In a cocktail shaker, combine tequila, lime juice, water, orange extract, allulose, erythritol or stevia, if using, and a small handful of ice. Shake until well blended. Alternatively, you can mix ingredients in a blender until slushy.
- If desired, wet the rim of a margarita or martini glass with lime juice or plain water and dip it into a small plate of margarita or kosher salt.
- Pour mixture from shaker into glass, either over ice or straight up. If blended, pour straight into glass.

Keto Cosmopolitan

Ingredients

1 jigger (1-½ ounces) vodka 1 ½ ounces or 3 tablespoons vodka

2 teaspoons unsweetened cranberry juice

2 tablespoons water

1 tablespoon lime juice fresh preferred

2 to 3 drops orange extract

1-2 teaspoons Swerve granulated

1 Lime wedge or lime peel for garnish

Instructions

- Add all ingredients to a cocktail shaker half-full of ice.
- Shake well.
- Taste for sweetness as unsweetened cranberry juice is highly variable. You may need to add more sweetener. Strain into a martini glass. Garnish with a small lime wedge or curl of lime peel.

Keto Mojito

Ingredients

8 mint leaves fresh

1-2 teaspoon swerve granulated

2 tbsp lime juice or lime wedges from about a third of a lime

1 jigger (1 ½ ounces) 80-proof white rum

Club soda

Garnish: fresh mint sprig

Instructions

- Put mint, a splash of club soda, and the swerve into the bottom of a highball glass or tall glass (if you like lots of ice and club soda). mash the ingredients together. If you have a muddler use that, otherwise the handle of a wooden spoon or spatula will work just fine.
- Squeeze the juice of the lime into the glass. Add the rum. Stir well.
- Fill the glass about ¾ of the way full with ice. Top off with club soda. Stir and enjoy. If serving in a tall glass, adding a cocktail straw is a useful touch.

Keto Moscow Mule

Ingredients

1 Jigger (1-½ oz) Vodka

½ oz (about ⅓ of a Jigger) Lime Juice

½ Cup Sugar free Zevia Ginger Beer

1 lime wedge for garnish

Ice

Instructions

- In a cocktail shaker add vodka, lime juice, ginger beer and ice.
- Shake lightly. Just enough to mix.
- Serve in a copper mug. Or if you don't have a copper mug a highball glass will work.

Notes

Some people add mint to these. You can do that if you want.

Keto Classic Daiquiri

Ingredients

2 ounces Rum either light or dark

1 teaspoon Swerve or to taste

1 ounce Lime Juice 1-2 Limes Squeezed

1 cup Ice

Instructions

- Put all of the ingredients in a cocktail shaker.
- Shake.
- Strain into a martini glass.
- Garnishe with a lime slice or one of those little umbrellas.

Enjoy

Notes

Some daiquiris call for a tablespoon of "simple syrup" instead of the teaspoon of swerve. If you would like to make your own zero carb simple syrup it is easy. Put ½ cup water and ½ cup of swerve in a sauce pan. Heat over medium heat. Stir slowly until swerve is completely dissolved.

Bourbon And Water

It does not get much easier than this mixed drink. Really, the name says it all: it's bourbon and water. It's also often called "bourbon and branch," referring to either the stream of water that flows into your bar glass or the branch of a river near a distillery.

While the question of how to make a bourbon and water is an easy one, a more pressing question is: When should you add water to your whiskey? Overall, it will be a personal preference. However, there are a few tips that can help guide you to get the most out of your whiskey.

Ingredients

2 ounces bourbon whiskey

1 splash mineral water

Steps to Make It

- Gather the ingredients.
- Pour the bourbon into an old-fashioned glass.
- Add a splash of water.
- Serve and enjoy.

Recipe Variations

- Alternatively, pour the whiskey over ice and allow it to melt a little bit before drinking.
- Some whiskey drinkers also enjoy a splash of soda water as seen in the popular Scotch and Soda.
- You might also enjoy your whiskey neat with a "water back." This extra glass of water allows you to either pour in a splash or two as you see fit or cleanse your palate after taking a straight sip.

Water Really Important

Bad water and good whiskey are a poor combination. Just like you (hopefully) will not fill your ice cube trays with standard tap water, it's important to think about the water you splash into your bourbon. The goal is to open up the whiskey's flavors, not pollute it with impurities.

Let's step back to the bourbon and branch moniker. "Branch water" is often used to refer to a branch of a water tributary that flows near a bourbon distillery. Some of the best bourbons are found in Kentucky because the water source flows through the natural filtration of limestone rock that dominates the region.

Iron is common in many unfiltered water sources and it will ruin a good bourbon. If you don't believe it, sacrifice a finger of bourbon and place a piece of iron in the glass. You will quickly see that it turns cloudy and gets a murky red hue. This is the chemical reaction of the iron and it's likely that your tap water contains some amount of the same mineral.

The limestone found in bourbon country naturally removes iron. However, there's no need to order up a truckload of Kentucky branch water for your whiskey. Mineral water, spring water, filtered water, and distilled water are all good choices. It doesn't matter which you choose as long as it's the cleanest water you have at your disposal. It seems like a trivial issue, but it's a simple step that will significantly improve your whiskey experience.

When To Add Water Or Ice To Whiskey

While the simple answer is to enjoy your whiskeys any way you like to drink them, there are a few suggestions for getting the most enjoyment out of your whiskey.

Whiskey Over 100 Proof

Cask-strength or barrel-proof whiskeys (usually those over 50 percent ABV, or 100 proof) can usually benefit from the addition of a splash of cool water or an ice cube or two. The flavors and aromas that might be missed in such a high-proof whiskey will begin to emerge and the burn of the alcohol becomes less noticeable.

If adding an ice cube, allow a few minutes for the whiskey and ice to warm up before drinking. As liquids become colder, less flavor is apparent. Adding a few cubes will actually tighten up the whiskey for a short time before the release of flavors becomes apparent.

90 Proof to 100 Proof Whiskey

Whiskeys that range from 45 percent to 50 percent ABV (90 to 100 proof) may be enhanced with water. Yet, you may also find that water detracts from your experience; it's going to depend on your palate and the whiskey in front of you.

Some whiskey drinkers find that a splash of water helps reduce the sting of alcohol while allowing them to detect subtle nuances in the spirit. Others find that the addition of water can make it feel thin and watery on their palate.

Professional tasters and reviewers often add a lot of water when reviewing whiskeys. This allows them to detect every flavor in a particular whiskey. They do this in the interest of their review, not to maximize their own enjoyment of the whiskey.

Trial and error are the only way to determine which method works best for you.

80 Proof Whiskey

Finally, whiskeys at 80 proof are probably best enjoyed neat. A whiskey at 40 percent ABV has already been cut down to this strength at the distillery and may not need additional water or ice.

This said, let your own palate be the ultimate arbiter of this discussion. Do not hesitate to order a whiskey on the rocks in a restaurant or bar if that is your preferred way to enjoy it.

Scotch And Soda

The name Scotch and soda tells you everything you need to know about this popular cocktail. While it is a very simple Scotch whisky drink, there are a few ways to improve it and customize it to suit your taste.

Adding still water to whisky opens up the liquor's flavor, and club soda will do the same. It also brings in a little effervescence to make it even more invigorating. The amount of soda is really up to you; some people prefer it in an old-fashioned glass while others like this drink as a highball. In terms of taste, a few ounces make a big difference: If you want a flavorful drink, go with a short pour of soda; for a softer drink, opt for the long pour.

The concept here is to water down Scotch without destroying the flavors of the whisky. In the process, you're making a longer-lasting, smoother, and more refreshing drink. Without a doubt, it's one of the easiest ways to dress up your favorite Scotch.

Ingredients

2 ounces Scotch whisky

1 to 6 ounces club soda, to taste

Steps to Make It

- Gather the ingredients
- In a highball or old-fashioned glass filled with ice, pour the Scotch.
- Scotch poured over ice

- Top with the club soda and stir well. Serve and enjoy.

Scotch and soda

Tips

- For the best Scotch and soda, be selective about which brand of soda you choose. A high-quality, craft club soda tends to have a cleaner profile and is a really nice complement to a decent Scotch.
- When serving it short, consider using an ice ball or large cube. These will melt slower than smaller cubes and prolong the drink's full flavor.

Recipe Variation

The two styles are very similar in taste, so switch from Scotch to Japanese whisky. In Japan, the highball drink is preferred. It's typically 1 1/2 ounces of whisky stirred with ice (often a long hand-carved cube) then topped with 4 to 5 ounces of soda.

From blended to single malts, any Scotch whisky can be used in a Scotch and soda, and it's a fantastic option when exploring new-to-you bottles. The beauty of this drink is that you can easily tailor it to fit the whisky you're pouring at the moment. For instance, when you have a great single malt, add just a splash of premium soda, but for a casual happy hour, choose an affordable blended whisky and fill a tall glass with soda.

Clear, unsweetened sodas are preferred in a Scotch and soda. Club soda is the easiest choice, though plain soda water out of a soda maker is excellent as well. Sparkling water tends to be less carbonated but is a good option. That said, ginger ale is commonly paired with whiskey in highballs, lemon-lime sodas add a sweet citrus spin, and Scotch and cola is a popular drink throughout Europe. Try different Scotches and other styles of whiskeys with various sodas to find your personal favorites for different moods.

Gin Martini

The classic dry gin martini is iconic and the world's most famous cocktail. Though many "martinis" have been created, there is only one true martini, and few drinks can beat this simple recipe. The flavor is a botanical bouquet with a dry profile that you can customize to your taste.

There is no mystery to the martini, and all you need to make one is your best gin and dry vermouth. There are countless ways to adjust the formula and technique: gin or vodka, dry or wet or dirty, shaken or stirred, olive or lemon garnish. All of these options have spurred a debate over the "proper" way to make a martini. While it's a never-ending discussion, the only correct answer is how you enjoy it. After all, you're drinking it.

Following some experimentation with this classic cocktail, you will know exactly how to make "the best martini" for your taste. Most of this will be adjusting the gin to vermouth ratio, exploring different brands, and choosing your preferred garnish. It's not a bad task to undertake, and you may even join the ranks of devoted martini connoisseurs.

Ingredients

2 1/2 ounces gin

1/2 ounce dry vermouth, or to taste

1 dash orange or aromatic bitters, optional

Lemon twist (or 1 or 3 olives), garnish

Steps to Make It

- Gather the ingredients Ingredients for a classic gin martini.
- In a mixing glass filled with ice cubes, combine the gin and vermouth, pouring more or less vermouth to your taste.
- Combine gin and vermouth in a mixing glass
- Stir for 30 seconds.
- Stirring the gin martini in the mixing glass
- Strain into a chilled cocktail glass.
- Pouring the gin martini into a chilled cocktail glass
- Add a dash of bitters, if desired.
- Adding a dash of orange bitters.
- Garnish with a lemon twist or olives.
- Classic gin martini garnished with olives on toothpicks

Tips

- The key to a great martini is to pour quality ingredients, so start off with a top-shelf gin and vermouth. With only two ingredients, this is not a cocktail where you want to be frugal.
- Every gin is different. You may want to change the ratio and the garnish when switching from one brand to another.
- Vermouth has a short shelf life because it's a fortified wine, not a distilled spirit. If your bottle has been open for longer than three months, it's time to replace it.

- It's thought that the lemon twist is the original martini garnish. The olives may have become an option when vodka was introduced as a gin substitute.
- For the olive garnish, skewer either one or three olives on a cocktail pick or simply drop them in the glass. It's an old bar tale that an even number of olives is bad luck.
- If the olives are big or stuffed with jalapeños, garlic, or the like, one olive will usually do. The flavor of the olive will slowly infuse into the drink and add just a little more dimension as it rests.

Recipe Variations

It's one drink, yet there are so many options. Among those are a few common recipes, and each has its own name:

Dry Martini: Traditionally, this used more dry vermouth, which seems like the most logical approach. However, today's dry martini is typically defined as using little or no vermouth; a "wet" martini uses more vermouth. Some drinkers will even simply wave a bottle of vermouth over the glass without adding a drop. It's said that Winston Churchill made his martinis by merely chilling gin and bowing in the direction of France, where dry vermouth originated.

Bone Dry or Desert Martini: Used for times when you want to clarify that no vermouth makes it into the mix. Essentially, you're drinking chilled gin.

50-50 Martini: The ultimate "wet" martini, this recipe uses equal parts of gin and dry vermouth.

Perfect Martini: Get a slightly sweeter profile by using equal parts of sweet and dry vermouth.

Vodka Martini: Replace the gin with vodka. This is popular among drinkers who don't necessarily enjoy the "piney flavor" of gin.

Gibson: Nothing changes from the original gin martini except the garnish. This cocktail makes use of those tiny cocktail onions.

Dirty Martini: Add a small amount of olive brine or juice to give the drink a salty-savory twist.

Good Times: An all-but-forgotten version, this classic mix uses 2 parts Old Tom gin and 1 part dry vermouth with a lemon twist.

Hanky Panky: Uses sweet vermouth and adds Fernet-Branca and orange juice.

Customizing The Martini

With all of the different approaches to the martini, it's fascinating to see how others prefer to mix it up. Over a nine-year period, The Spruce Eats did an informal poll to see how drinkers take their martinis, and the results are rather interesting.

Of the 90,000 people who responded, over half (59 percent) preferred gin over vodka. The overwhelming majority of those drinkers enjoy a full dose of vermouth, and only 13 percent prefer little or no vermouth.

Whether it includes gin or vodka, there was a slim majority (52 percent) who shake their martinis. Only 39 percent opted for the traditional stir; everyone else prefers to skip the martini altogether. This is interesting considering the classic advice regarding when to shake or stir cocktails. In general, bartenders stir liquor-only drinks, saving the shake for more complex and mixer-heavy cocktails.

The traditional options are not your only choices. Many martini fans put their personal spin on preparing it. Chilling one or both bottles in the refrigerator is among the most common, and some use the freezer. This ensures that the gin and vermouth are always cold and lets you avoid any dilution from ice.

That approach will produce the most flavorful martini possible, and it is a very nice drink. However, without dilution, the drink will remain at the bottling proof and may be too strong for some people. As an extra benefit, the small amount of water relaxes the drink and marries the botanical flavors. Shaking the martini with ice adds more dilution and further softens the taste. This may explain why many drinkers prefer that approach.

Wine Spritzer

Wine spritzers are lovely little wine-based drinks that feature a splash of sweet soda and taste summery fresh. Wine spritzers were undoubtedly the inspiration for the wine coolers of the late 80s and early 90s. While not a novel concept, they are enjoyed in many wine-producing regions under different names. In Germany, for example, this cocktail is dubbed "süssgespritzter", referring to wine or cider mixed with lemonade or a citrus-inspired soda. On the canals of Venice, Italians enjoy a spritz Veneziano (or, simply, "spreetz"), a refreshing combination of sparkling wine, Aperol (an Italian orange liqueur), and soda water. The French 75, created in France around World War I, mixes champagne with gin, simple syrup, and lemon juice.

A wine spritzer is perfect when you have a bottle of white, red, or rosé wine on hand and the temperature outside is balmy. The ice and soda turn what could be too heavy a drink for summer into a refreshing cocktail that is not only cooling but also lower in alcohol strength not a bad idea when the heat is on. Turn it up a notch and add some fresh seasonal fruit to your glass.

Ingredients

4 ounces ice

3 ounces wine (white, red, or rose)

3 ounces soda (citrus flavors are great)

Optional: seasonal fruit

Steps to Make It

- Gather the ingredients easy Wine Spritzer ingredients.
- Fill an 8-ounce tumbler halfway with ice.
- Add the wine and soda to the ice in the glass.
- Toss in slices of your favorite fruit, if desired.
- add the fruit to the wine spritzer
- Stir and enjoy.

Best Wine For Wine Spritzers

When choosing a wine to make wine spritzers, the most important characteristic is that you enjoy drinking it on its own; if you would not pour a glass to sip at cocktail hour or with dinner, then don't use it in this recipe (in fact, you probably shouldn't use it in anything where you will taste the wine); bad or unpleasant tasting wine won't get any better when mixed with soda and ice. But if you are selecting a bottle just for the purpose of making a spritzer, reach for something that has a good fruity flavor and mild tannins; Sauvignon Blanc, Riesling, and Pinot Noir are all great choices.

Other Wine-Based Cocktails

If you find yourself with a few bottles of wine but are looking for more interesting ways to serve and drink them, there are many refreshing recipes that combine vino with other ingredients to make party-worthy cocktails. There is sangria, of course, which can take on a variety of flavors depending on the type of fruit you add. A strawberry-lime sangria is ideal for summer, with a blend of rose, lemon-lime soda, fresh strawberries, and mint, while citrus sangria brings together grapefruit, orange, lemon, and lime for a refreshing cocktail on a warm day.

But there are also some perhaps lesser-known wine-based recipes worth trying, like a bishop cocktail, a mixture of red wine, rum, simple syrup, and lime juice, and a glamour girl martini, which combines rose, peach schnapps, and cranberry juice.

Pickleback Shot

The pickleback is a very interesting whiskey shot and a drink you have to experience for yourself. It's incredibly simple a shot of Jameson chased by a shot of pickle juice and it is, without a doubt, one of the most popular shots ordered in bars around the world.

Chasing whiskey with pickle brine really is nothing new; it's long been one of those "hair of the dog" remedies for hangovers. Yet, it wasn't until 2006 that Brooklyn bartender Reggie Cunningham gave the shot its now-famous name at the Bushwick Country Club. After that, it didn't take long for the drink to become a hit and spread across the U.S. and beyond.

The combination is odd, though it works surprisingly well. Even if you're not a fan of pickles, it's a drink you'll want to try because it delivers a rich, umami flavor that you will not find in any other drink. There's no need to head to the bar, either. You can experience the pickleback at home, even with that jar of Vlasic pickles hanging out in your fridge.

Ingredients

1 1/2 ounces Irish whiskey, like Jameson

1 1/2 ounces pickle juice

Steps to Make It

- Gather the Ingredients for pickleback shot.

- Pour one shot glass full of whiskey and fill a separate shot glass with pickle juice.
- Pouring pickle juice into a shot glass

Tip

Many people have found that a beer chaser is a perfect way to finish up the pickleback, though it's not required. If you'd like to give it a try, stick with the light, refreshing lagers. Dos Equis, Tecate, and Pabst Blue Ribbon are some of the top choices among pickleback fans.

The Irish Whiskey

The key to making a great pickleback really is in the whiskey. You can pour any Irish whiskey or any other whiskey, for that matter but it will not be the same as a shot of Jameson. Maybe it's this particular whiskey's woody sweetness or something else entirely. It's hard to explain why, but Jameson creates the best tasting pickleback.

While Jameson is not the original whiskey, it is the most popular today, and likely led to the shot's success. Cunningham's first round (or 10 rounds, according to his account) of the pickleback actually used Old Crow. This is good news if you want a pickleback and want to save money. It's not quite as tasty as Jameson, but it's pretty good.

The Pickle Juice

As stringent as you should be about the whiskey, there's no need to be picky about the pickle juice. The brine from any jar of pickles will work. Go ahead and pour from that commercially produced jar or your favorite homemade pickles the shot will be just as good either way.

The pickle juice is also where you can have some fun. Bartenders around the country have played with a variety of pickle bases to great success. Some bars even stock up to 10 jars for this exact purpose. Try fruity brines, spicy brines, or something in between to see which you like best. If you want to keep it authentic, McClure's is the brand of pickles Cunningham used and recommends.

Vodka Collins Cocktail

The vodka collins is a simple, refreshing, and popular mixed drink. Made with vodka, lemon juice, simple syrup, and club soda, it's really just a sweet and sour vodka soda (and just as easy to mix up). The quick but charming cocktail is a perfect happy hour choice for vodka drinkers, and its clean, crisp taste makes it ideal for dinner.

This recipe follows the formula common in the collins family of drinks: spirit, sour, sweet, soda. It's nearly identical to the Tom Collins (gin) and the John Collins (whiskey) and simply uses vodka as the base spirit. If you want to stick with proper names, this recipe is also called a Joe Collins, though that name is rarely used.

While almost any vodka will do, this drink is rather transparent. It will only be as good as the liquor you pour there's no way to hide a less-than-stellar vodka choice. That said, you don't have to overthink this. Any of the popular premium vodkas are good options. Choose wisely when it comes to budget-friendly vodkas; they're not all worthy of clear drinks like the vodka collins.

Ingredients

1 1/2 ounces vodka

1 ounce lemon juice

1/2 ounce simple syrup

3 to 5 ounces club soda, to taste

Orange slice, garnish

Maraschino cherry, garnish

Steps to Make It

- Gather the ingredients for vodka Collins
- In a collins glass filled with ice cubes, pour the vodka, lemon juice, and simple syrup. Stir thoroughly.
- Liquids poured into a Collins glass with ice
- Top with club soda.
- Club soda poured on top of vodka
- Garnish with a orange slice and cherry. Serve and enjoy.

Tips

- Fresh-squeezed lemon juice is highly recommended. Half of the average lemon should yield enough juice for one drink.
- Adjust the sweet and sour proportions to find the taste that best suits you.

Recipe Variations

Add a splash of flavor by switching to your favorite flavored vodka. Any fruit flavor works well, though it's not the best drink for whipped cream and other sweet vodkas.

Eliminate the lemon juice and simple syrup and use 1 1/2 ounces of a homemade sour mix instead. Limoncello is another interesting substitute for the two ingredients.

Give the vodka collins an herbal twist by infusing the syrup with herbs. Lavender, mint, or rosemary syrup are all excellent choices.

For a sugar-free cocktail, skip the sweetener and enjoy a lemon-kissed vodka soda or switch to sugar-free syrup.

Try the ultra-refreshing cucumber collins with cucumber, lime, and mint.

The almost a collins is filled with flavor, mixing blood orange juice and soda with cinnamon syrup.

Separator Cocktail

If you replace the vodka of a black Russian with brandy you have this drink called a brandy separator. It's an equally pleasant drink and you can add cream to make a white brandy seperator.

All of these drinks are connected and very easy to remember. This brandy version is just as good, if not better than the vodka drink and it is a great cold weather cocktail.

Ingredients

1 1/2 ounces brandy

3/4 ouncecoffee liqueur

Steps to Make It

- Gather the ingredients.
- Ingredients for a Separator Cocktail With Brandy and Coffee Liqueur
- Build the ingredients in an old-fashioned glass with ice cubes.
- Mixing a Separator Cocktail with Brandy and Coffee Liqueur
- Stir well.
- Mixing a Separator Cocktail With Brandy and Coffee Liqueur
- Serve and enjoy.

Recipe Variation

To make a white brandy separator, mix 1 1/2 ounce brandy and 1/2 ounce coffee liqueur in an old-fashioned glass over ice. Float cream on top to fill.

Lemon Drop Martini

The lemon drop is one of the best vodka martinis and a highlight of modern cocktail menus. Created by San Francisco bartender Norman Jay Hobday in the 1970s, it became so popular that it inspired a number of ready-to-drink variations. However, the recipe is very easy and there's no need for a mix the fresh taste is far better than any bottled lemon drop can offer.

Like many of the best cocktails, the lemon drop requires just a few ingredients. You'll choose your favorite vodka and shake that with lemon juice and simple syrup. Quite often, the lemon drop is served with a sugar rim. With each sip, the sweetness is a brilliant introduction to the sweet and sour drink and it's reminiscent of sugar-coated lemon drop candies.

This is a great dessert drink and a fabulous choice when you want a cocktail with a bit of pucker and a hint of sweetness. You can also adapt it to suit your personal taste and have fun adding other flavors to the mix.

Click Play to See This Easy and Fresh Lemon Drop Martini Recipe Come Together

Ingredients

Granulated sugar, for rimming

Lemon wedge, for rimming

2 ounces vodka

1 ounce freshly squeezed lemon juice, from 1 lemon

1/2 to 3/4 ounce simple syrup, to taste

Lemon twist, garnish

Steps to Make It

- Gather the ingredients.
- Rim a cocktail glass with sugar: Place the sugar in a shallow dish. Wipe a lemon wedge around the glass to wet the surface, then dip it into the sugar. Set aside to dry while you mix the drink.
- Rim the cocktail glass with sugar
- In a cocktail shaker filled with ice, pour the vodka, lemon juice, and simple syrup.
- ice, vodka, lemon juice, and simple syrup in a cocktail shaker
- Shake well.
- Shake the cocktail shaker
- Strain into the rimmed glass.
- strain the cocktail into a sugar rimmed glass
- Garnish with a lemon twist. Serve and enjoy.
- Lemon Drop Martini, garnished with a lemon twist

Tips

Simple drinks like this deserve and almost require the best ingredients. The foundation is vodka, so begin building the best tasting cocktail possible by choosing a smooth vodka. There are many fantastic premium vodkas perfect for cocktails of this caliber. If your budget is tight, you can also find some nice inexpensive vodkas.

To get the absolute best lemon drop, the lemon juice and syrup should both be fresh. One lemon will yield enough juice for one or two drinks and homemade syrup is easy to make.

If you find the drink to be a little too tart, add more syrup next time. Likewise, if it's a bit too sweet for your taste, pour more lemon juice.

Variations

Add extra flavor with citrus or another fruit vodka.

A fun addition, 1/2 ounce of limoncello gives the lemon drop an extra sweetened lemon flavor.

Fruit syrups are simple to make and berries are a nice pairing for the tart lemon juice.

Floral syrups can also add a fun twist. For instance, a lavender simple syrup creates a lovely lavender lemon drop martini. In spring, get a similar flavor by harvesting lilac blooms for a lilac lemon drop martini.

Another simple variation adds 1/4 ounce Cointreau and uses only 1/2 teaspoon simple syrup. This brings in an orange undertone that complements the sweetened lemon.

If you're in the mood for a shot, try the lemon drop shot. It has the same great flavor in an interactive shooter that's quite fun.

How to Make Your Own Lemon Drop Martini Mix

Lemon drop martini mixes are, essentially, a lemon sour sweetened lemon juice in a convenient pour-and-shake package. You can replicate that by making a fresh lemon sour at home: Replace the lime juice in a standard sour mix recipe with lemon juice.

The advantage of pouring lemon juice and simple syrup separately is that you can adjust the sweet and sour to taste. You can still get that customization in a homemade lemon sour: Take notes while mixing up the martini with the individual ingredients until you find an ideal balance. Use that sweet-sour ratio when making your lemon sour and bottle it. This makes it even easier to enjoy a lemon drop anytime you like because you simply need to add vodka and shake it up.

How To Create The Lemon Twist Garnish

The lemon twist is one of the trickiest citrus garnishes to cut. It's not difficult, but it does take a little practice.

Use a canelle knife or sharp paring knife and hold the whole lemon firmly in one hand.

Dig the knife into the peel, just deep enough to avoid most of the white pith.

In a smooth motion, roll the fruit in your hand as the knife cuts a thin strip of peel. You can stop whenever it reaches the desired length or when it naturally cuts off.

Roll the peel into a tight spiral and gently squeeze it without breaking the peel. The twist will loosen up once released; keep it in a glass of ice water to maintain a nice spiral.

Keto Hot Chocolate

Warming and sweet wintry beverages are beloved by nearly everyone people looking to avoid sugar or following a ketogenic diet. It's wonderful to whip up a fresh mug every time you have the urge for a steaming mug of cocoa, but it's even more delightful to have a healthful homemade mix on hand that renders sugar-free hot chocolate a quick moment away at any time. We've created a keto hot chocolate mix that keeps indefinitely in a jar or container and needs only hot water added to be enjoyed one toasty cup at a time.

The secret to making a hot chocolate mix that's low in carbs is powdered coconut milk. Containing no ingredients beyond the tinned version, it's made from just coconut and a minimal amount of tapioca starch or acacia gum for thickening and weighs in at three carbs or less per serving. Powdered coconut milk is available at health food stores, some mainstream groceries, and online from sites like Amazon and Thrive Market. Another option is "superfood creamer," which is powdered coconut milk that has dried coconut oil added. The coconut oil will give a richer taste, so it's a good option if you want a hot chocolate that is more indulgent.

This keto hot chocolate can be enjoyed plain, amped up with some heavy cream or full-fat coconut milk, made extra chocolatey with sugar-free chocolate chips melted in, or with one of our many flavor variations below.

Ingredients

1 cup granular keto sweetener (such as allulose or monkfruit)

1/2 cup cocoa powder

1/2 cup powdered coconut milk

1/4 teaspoon salt

Steps to Make It

- Gather all the ingredients for keto hot chocolate.
- Mix all the ingredients, keto sweetener, cocoa powder, powdered coconut milk, and salt, in a mixing bowl with a whisk until uniform in texture.
- Dry ingredients whisked together in small bowl.
- Pour into a mason jar or plastic food-storage container and seal tightly.
- Dry hot chocolate ingredients in jar
- When ready to use, add 2 tablespoons hot chocolate mix to a mug and add 10 ounces of very hot water. Stir well.
- Keto hot chocolate in mug with some mix on the side

Tip

When stored in a tightly-sealed container, this hot cocoa mix will last for six months.

Recipe Variations

There are many ways that this hot chocolate can be made even more wintry and fun! Because some flavorings are liquid-based, proportions offered here are on a by-the-cup basis. If there's a spice you love that holds up well in storage, such as cinnamon, chipotle, or nutmeg, feel free to add it directly to the batch of mixing when whisking it up initially and avoid conflicting flavor choices below.

Below are some festive ways to enhance the cocoa one cup at a time; add any of the combos to the mix in the cup, just before pouring the hot water over it.

Peppermint

1/2 teaspoon peppermint extract (or 1/4 teaspoon peppermint stevia for an extra kick of sweetness)

1/4 teaspoon vanilla extract

Mexican Hot Chocolate:

1/2 teaspoon cinnamon

1/8 teaspoon nutmeg

1/4 teaspoon vanilla

Optional: 1/8 teaspoon chipotle powder

Orange:

1/2 tablespoon grated orange zest

1/4 teaspoon orange extract

Nutty:

1/4 teaspoon almond extract

1/4 teaspoon hazelnut stevia

Sticky Sweet:

1/2 teaspoon caramel extract

1/2 teaspoon toffee stevia

Mocha:

1/2 teaspoon coffee extract

1/4 teaspoon vanilla extract

Pumpkin Spice:

1/2 teaspoon pumpkin pie spice

1 teaspoon pumpkin puree

1 teaspoon sugar-free "maple syrup"

Coconut:

1 to 2 teaspoons MCT or coconut oil

Keto Eggnog

Eggnog enjoys such a quick season in grocery stores that people often rush to stock up on the sweet, creamy holiday drink. However, if you follow a keto diet or you don't want to consume a lot of sugar in a single cup, the store-bought versions won't work for you. Thankfully, making scrumptious and festive keto eggnog isn't complex!

In this keto eggnog recipe, you'll make a basic custard that's similar to an ice cream base. It uses the traditional preparation method and flavors, like nutmeg and cinnamon, that you expect from eggnog but without any of the sugar. The result is keto eggnog with all the tastes and textures you know and love.

To transform traditional eggnog into a keto beverage, this recipe replaces the sweetener and milk. For the sweetener, the sugar is swapped out for a combination of confectioner's Swerve (an erythritol-based sweetener) and liquid stevia. Instead of milk, the recipe uses unsweetened almond milk, and other plant-based milks work well too. Because it uses heavy cream, which is fully keto, the swap from dairy milk isn't nearly as noticeable as it would be if cream weren't involved.

Serve the eggnog as is or spike it with alcohol by the glass. For a festive touch, dust the drinks with nutmeg and add a cinnamon stick garnish.

Ingredients

5 egg yolks

1/4 cup confectioners' Swerve

2 cups unsweetened almond milk

1 1/4 cups heavy cream

1/2 teaspoon cinnamon

1/2 teaspoon ground nutmeg

1/2 teaspoon liquid stevia

1 teaspoon rum extract

1 teaspoon vanilla extract

Steps to Make It

- Gather the ingredients of Keto Eggnog.
- In a medium-sized mixing bowl, whisk the egg yolks with powdered Swerve until light and frothy. Set aside once whisked.
- Whisk egg yolks with powdered Swerve in a bowl
- In a medium-sized saucepan, add the almond milk, cream, cinnamon, and nutmeg and turn the heat to medium-high. Bring to a boil, then immediately remove the mixture from the heat.
- Add the almond milk, cream, cinnamon, and nutmeg in a saucepan
- Slowly pour half of the heated milk, cream, and spice mixture in a thin stream over the egg yolk and Swerve mixture while whisking constantly and quickly. This is most easily done with a mixing cup or ladle to make sure you don't add it too quickly.
- Pour half of the heated milk, cream, and spice mixture in a thin stream over the egg yolk

- Pour the tempered egg and milk mixture back into the pot with the remaining milk, cream, and spices, continuing to whisk vigorously. Turn the heat to medium-low.
- Pour the tempered egg and milk mixture back into the pot with the remaining milk, cream, and spices
- Continue whisking as the mixture cooks and thickens, lowering the heat to low if it nears boiling. It will take about 7 minutes and should be approximately 160 F when cooked.
- Cook the eggnog in the pot
- Remove the eggnog from the heat and add the stevia and extracts, whisking them to incorporate. Pour eggnog through a mesh strainer to remove any lumps, then refrigerate until cold, about 2 hours.
- Add stevia and extracts to the Keto Eggnog in the pot

Raw Egg Warning

Consuming raw and lightly-cooked eggs poses a risk of food-borne illness.

Tips

Room temperature egg yolks will whip up more easily than cold ones straight from the fridge.

Because erythritol can crystallize when heated, we don't recommend using a different brand, specifically if it doesn't have the additional ingredients contained in Swerve that prevent crystallization.

The eggnog may thicken further as it cools. If the chilled drink is too thick for you, thin it out 1 tablespoon at a time with almond milk before serving.

Eggnog can be stored in a sealed container for up to three days in the refrigerator.

Recipe Variations

Substitute the almond milk for unsweetened flax or coconut boxed milk instead if you prefer the taste.

To avoid dairy altogether, substitute the heavy cream with full-fat coconut milk. Take care to add it at the end, and not to boil it, as it's prone to separating. This means you'll bring the almond milk and spices to a boil alone, and add the coconut milk when along with the stevia and extracts after cooking the eggnog, just before straining.

If you plan on mixing this eggnog with alcohol, you can omit the rum extract. Brandy, rum, and whiskey are best with eggnog; add about 1 1/2 ounces to a glass of eggnog and stir well.

For most people, eggnog is safe to drink. The USDA states that youth, older adults, and pregnant women are most susceptible to food poisoning from consuming raw or lightly cooked eggs.1There are ways to reduce the risks in any drink that includes eggs: Choose undamaged pasteurized eggs in the shell from refrigerated cases, refrigerate them promptly when you get home, and check that the eggs are still fresh before separating them safely.

Most people enjoy eggnog cold, though some prefer it warm. Taste it for yourself before refrigerating the keto eggnog to see what you think. It doesn't reheat well, so it's best to make a batch just before serving if you find it more enjoyable warm.

Low-Carb Raspberry & Blackberry Mojitos

INGREDIENTS

The Mojito is a great addition to keto cocktails. It can be given a summer twist by adding fresh raspberries and blackberries. Blueberries will be fine too. It has a total carb amount of 4.6g.

1/2 cup raspberries and/or blackberries (70 g/ 2.5 oz)

1/2 cup loosely packed mint

4 tbsp fresh lime juice (60 ml/ 2 fl oz)

4 tbsp powdered Erythritol or Swerve or 10-20 drops liquid stevia (Sweet

Leaf or NuNaturals) or 1 -2 tbsp Sukrin Clear Syrup

1/2 cup white rum (120 ml/ 4 fl oz)

ice cubes

1 cup sparkling water (club soda) or as needed to top up (240 ml/ 8 fl oz)

INSTRUCTION

Place the raspberries (or blackberries), lime juice, mint and powdered Erythritol in 2 tall glasses. Few berries can be kept to g arnish.Crush the berries using a long spoon or a muddler and muddle the mint leaves to extract flavor.

Pour in white rum

Add ice and top up with sparkling water (club soda).

Finally, garnish with more mint leaves, lime wedges and berries.

Low Carb Margaritas

Prepari ng this cocktail does not entail much since the best margaritas are very simple with no fancy or added ingredients. You can choose to take it blended or on the rocks. It contains a total carb of 3g.

INGREDIENTS

3 ounces good tequila white

2 ounces freshly squeezed lime juice

1/2 tsp orange extract

1 tbsp powdered Swerve Sweetener optional

Crushed ice

Kosher salt for rimming optional

INSTRUCTION

In a cocktail shaker or a measuring cup, combine tequila, lime juice, orange extract and sweetener, if using.

Fill two margarita glasses or old-fashioned glasses halfway with crushed ice.

Divide mixture evenly between glasses.

If you like a salted rim, run a wedge of lime around the outside of the glass before filling with ice and dip in a plate of kosher salt.

Low Carb Moscow Mules

For the Moscow Mule:

4 oz premium vodka

1 oz fresh lime juice

This is a low carb vodka cocktail flavored with ginger, lime and mint. It has 1.5g of carb.

INGREDIENTS

For the Ginger Syrup:

1/2 cup thinly sliced, peeled ginger

2 cups water

1/3 cup granulated sugar substitute

1 oz ginger syrup (recipe above)8 oz diet ginger ale

fresh mint leaves to garnish

INSTRUCTIONS

For the Ginger Syrup:

Combine the ginger, water and sweetener in a small saucepan.

Bring to a boil over high heat. Lower the heat to medium and simmer for 10

minutes.

Cool for 1 hour, then strain and store in a clean jar in the fridge for up to 2

weeks.

For the Moscow Mules:

Combine the vodka, lime juice, ginger syrup and ginger ale in a small pitcher.

Stir well.

Pour over ice and garnish with fresh mint. For a stronger mint flavor, muddle

(smash) the mint leaves around in the bottom of the mug slightly before drinking.

Low Carb Sparkling Sangria

This refreshing low carb sangria recipe has all of the flavor of the real thing, without the sugar and carbs. It is keto friendly at only 50 calories and 1 net carb per serving.

INGREDIENTS

be used) 1/2 cup pureed fresh or frozen peaches

1/4 cup Torani sugar free mango flavored syrup 1/4 cup bourbon

1/2 cup vodka

2 Tbsp granulated sugar substitute (Swerve can also

1 Tbsp lime juice

24 oz (2 cans) mandarin flavored seltzer water

INSTRUCTION

Combine all of the ingredients in a large pitcher and stir well.Garnish with raspberries and/or slices of fresh peach if desired.Serve over ice.

Vanilla Old-Fashioned

INSTRUCTIONS

This is another suitable and keto-friendly cocktail with 3g of carbs.

INGREDIENTS

0.25 oz. Simple Syrup

3 dashes Angostura Bitters

3 dashes Orange Bitters

Orange Peel Twist

1.5 oz. vanilla whiskey

In old-fashioned glass, combine simple syrup and bitters.

Fill glass halfway with ice, then stir.

Add enough ice to fill glass.

Squeeze orange peel over glass to extract oils, add peel to glass, and add whiskey.

Stir just until drink is cold and serve.

BREAKDOWN OF HOW TO MAKE A SIMPLE SYRUP

Empty Equal Volume of Water And Sugar In A Saucepan

Since it is an established fact that sugar dissolves into the water, therefore 1 cup of sugar and 1 cup of water will not give 2 cups of simple syrup. Hence, you should expect 1½ cups of simple syrup from 1 cup of sugar and 1 cup of water when dissolved.

Cook/Heat the Ingredients Until Dissolved

Place the simple syrup in a saucepan over medium heat after mixing. By the time the edges start to simmer, the liquid should be completely clear. Then remove from the heat source.

Add flavor

If you are making infused simple syrups, you can then add the extra ingredients. Stir them into the syrup immediately it comes off the burner and cover to allow the simple syrup to steep. Different flavors of simple syrup can be achieved by pouring the liquid into jars with different ingredients. Cover the jars with the lids while steeping.

Remove Additional Ingredients Once the Simple Syrup Is Cool

Never leaving mint leaves or citrus rind in the simple syrup long -term as this will only shorten its shelf life. If you're creating a cocktail bar, you can always garnish the simple syrups later with another cinnamon stick or sprig of rosemary.

Keep It Cold

Ensure the simple syrup is contained in an airtight container and kept in the fridge until ready to use. Basic simple syrup can stay fresh up to 4 weeks, however flavored simple syrups must be used within a week or two.

The Green Tox Cocktail

INSTRUCTIONS

The green juice can be used in this drink. It has been a staple since Las Vegas' Honey Salt opened. This recipe can be made in no time and it has a low carb of 15g. It can be garnished with lemon wheel.

INGREDIENTS

1 1/2 oz Tito's Handmade vodka

2 oz Green goodness juice

3/4 oz Agave nectar

1 splash Fresh lemon juice

Add all the ingredients into a shaker with ice, and shake until well-chilled. Strain into a rocks glass over fresh ice.

Garnish with a lemon wheel.

Low Carb Kamikaze Shot

INGREDIENTS

3/4 shaker Ice

2 tbsp Lime Juice

You can also enjoy this sugary party pleaser in a low carb form. All you need do is get a low carb sweetener like Erythritol or Stevia in place of the triple sec and syrup. 2g of carbs is obtainable from this cocktail.

2 g Granulated Stevia or Erythritol

1 shot Vodka

INSTUCTIONS

Place ice in shaker.

Add lime juice, sweetener, and vodka.Cover and shake.

Serve in chilled rocks glass or short tumbler.

Red Wine Berry Spritzer

Red wine berry spritzer is one great keto -friendly cocktail which is really just a combo of red wine and berry-flavored seltzer water, topped with ice and frozen berries. Super easy and tasty, without any added sugar.

Spritzers are a great low -calorie cocktail, since seltzer water is calorie-free, and they're especially great for those who dislike the bitterness of red wine. Originally, I thought they would need a little added sweetness, but surprisingly the berry seltzer added
enough flavor that you don't need any extra sugar.

INGREDIENTS

½ cup wine

½ cup berry-flavored seltzer water

Frozen berries

INSTRUCTIONS

Fill a wine or cocktail glass with ice.

Pour wine into glass until halfway full, then fill remaining glass with seltzer water and stir.

Garnish with frozen berries.

Low Carb Lemon Drop Martini

INSTRUCTIONS

This cocktail can also be enjoyed while maintaining your keto diet. It contains 4g of carbs.

INGREDIENTS

1 1/2 ounces lemon vodka

2 ounces fresh lemon juice

Pinch sugar, or baking stevia, optional

2 ounces plain or lemon sparkling water, such as La Croix

1 lemon wedge

Sugar for rimming

Rim the top of a martini glass with the lemon wedge. And dip into sugar to coat. Set aside.

In a shaker, add the lemon vodka, lemon juice, stevia if using and a handful of ice. Shake for 15 seconds. Strain into martini glass, leaving the ice in the shaker. Top with sparkling water.

Serve immediately.

Grapefruit Ginger Fizz

1/2 cup swerve

zest of one grapefruit

1 teaspoon of grated gingerDrink

1 oz of gin or vodka

2 Tablespoons of fresh grapefruit juice

1 teaspoon of syrup

Gingerale to taste

INSTRUCTIONS

In a saucepan, add your water, ginger, grapefruit zest and swerve.Simmer until all the Swerve has melted, set to low and let sit for 5 minutes.Take off the burner and let cool.

In a drinking glass, add vodka or gin, grapefruit juice and 1 teaspoon of syrup. Add gingerale to taste.

Please note you will have enough syrup for quite a few drinks. This grapefruit ginger fizz cocktail is a tasty low carb drink for Spring. Fresh grapefruit juice coupled with spicy ginger for a refreshing cocktail. Tastes great with either vodka or gin. 2.8g of carbs is obtainable per drink.

INGREDIENTS

Syrup

1/2 cup water